YOGA NIDRA SCRIPTS

Write your own sessions with ease

Valerie Saier

Independent

ISBN: 9798860497290

Contributor: Eva Afentouli

CONTENTS

BRIEF HISTORY OF YOGA NIDRA

Yoga Nidra's origins can be traced back to ancient India, where it emerged as a meditative practice within the tantric tradition. The Sanskrit word "nidra" translates to sleep, but in this context, it refers to a state of consciousness that lies between wakefulness and sleep.

Traditionally, Yoga Nidra was practiced to delve into the profound layers of the mind, accessing inner wisdom, and experiencing spiritual insights. In Western contexts, it is more often seen and use as a means of relaxation and stress reduction.

The modern form of Yoga Nidra was developed in the mid-20th century by Swami Satyananda Saraswati, the founder of the Bihar School of Yoga in India, and the author of the book "Yoga Nidra". He systematized the practice, combining different techniques in a specific order. His book contributed to the global popularity of Yoga Nidra beyond India, making it accessible to a diverse range of individuals.

Today, Yoga Nidra is practiced worldwide to induce relaxation, mitigate stress, and deepen spiritual exploration.

UNDERSTANDING YOGA NIDRA SCRIPTS

Unlike meditation, Yoga Nidra is always practiced under the verbal guidance of a live or recorded instructor. The guidance is conveyed through Yoga Nidra scripts, which come in myriad variations.

Numerous books and websites provide pre-written Yoga Nidra scripts catering to a diverse array of themes. However, if you aim to inspire transformation and help your clients navigate their unique challenges, it's advisable to develop the skill of crafting your own scripts.

Because Yoga Nidra is a blend of different techniques, it is advisable to maintain certain guidelines for scripts writing. These guidelines ensure that your practice remains authentic to Yoga Nidra's essence, safeguarding it from being mistaken for mere relaxation, visualization, or dreaming. Remember, Yoga Nidra is a state of heightened consciousness.

In the upcoming sections, we will delve deeper into the components of Yoga Nidra scripts for a more comprehensive understanding.

Purpose of Yoga Nidra Scripts

Yoga Nidra scripts serve as a guiding framework for practitioners to enter into a state of profound relaxation and attain a state of heightened awareness. These scripts skillfully lead individuals from the outer layers of consciousness to the most subtle realms within. Acting as a navigational map, the script offers clear instructions, while allowing room for personalization and adaptability.

Anatomy of a Yoga Nidra Script

A Yoga Nidra script is composed of distinct stages that progress from the external to the internal. Each stage encompasses specific directives for the practitioner to follow, with some stages being mandatory while others are optional.

Types of Yoga Nidra Scripts

There are many different types of Yoga Nidra scripts, each with its own focus. Some are designed to alleviate stress, while others focus on improving the quality of sleep. Others lean towards spiritual exploration, while some adopt a more secular approach. Scripts may be tailored for specific demographics, such as children or pregnant women. However, it is crucial to bear in mind that the essence of Yoga Nidra revolves around liberating ourselves from the grip of subconscious patterns.

Common Elements in Yoga Nidra Scripts

Although individual Yoga Nidra scripts vary, certain common elements frequently emerge. These elements encompass a relaxation phase, a comprehensive body scan, breath awareness, guided visualization, and a gradual re-emergence into waking consciousness. These components collectively contribute to the holistic experience of Yoga Nidra, facilitating relaxation, self-awareness, and inner transformation.

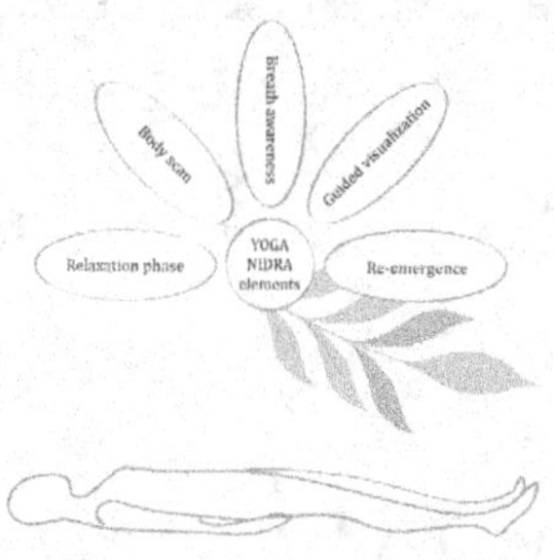

YOGA NIDRA & KOSHAS PATH

As we have discussed, embarking on a journey without guidelines is akin to traveling without a roadmap. While you might eventually reach your destination, there's no certainty. To ensure a timely and fulfilling journey, meticulous preparation becomes essential. You set stepping stones (guide lines) to follow, enabling you to cover the distance you've envisioned.

Likewise, I recommend using the Panchamaya Kosha system as the foundational framework for your Yoga Nidra script.

The 5 Koshas

The Panchamaya Koshas comprise five interwoven layers enveloping Pure Consciousness. Those sheaths are interdependent and represent different dimensions of being. Those 5 koshas can serve as a roadmap for our voyage of self-discovery. By delving into and harmonizing each layer, we advance towards heightened awareness and self-realization.

1st sheath: Annamaya Kosha - The outermost layer, which literally means "food sheath". It corresponds to the physical body.

It encompasses matter, including skin, bones, muscles, organs, and tissues. Through Annamaya Kosha, we engage with the physical world and interface with the natural surroundings.

2d sheath: Pranamaya Kosha - The energy sheath, composed of the five major pranas, facilitates the flow of life force energy. Pranamaya Kosha plays a pivotal role in vital functions.

3d sheath: Manomaya Kosha - The mental sheath incorporates emotions, thoughts, feelings, memories, and imagination. It is where we process our experiences and emotions. It governs cognitive functions like memory, perception, and reasoning.

4th sheath: Vijnanamaya Kosha - The intellect sheath encompasses intuition, intellect, and inner wisdom. This kosha fosters our connection with the inner self and the universe. Here lies our ability to discern right from wrong and real from illusion, making it a key factor in our spiritual evolution.

5th sheath: Anandamaya Kosha - The bliss-filled sheath, the finest veil enveloping the Self (atman), often known as the level of the soul. It enables us feelings joy, love, happiness, spiritual contentment, and liberation. It fosters our interconnectedness with all existence.

Keeping in mind that the purpose of Yoga Nidra practices guide us toward discovering the infinite within, an unbounded space where we experience fulfillment and connection with our True Self. Seeing how the kosha path goes from the external to the internal, from the material to the non-material, from the physical to the spiritual. We can understand that this path aptly mirrors the mechanics of a Yoga Nidra script and that using this pattern ensures that practitioners traverse progressively inward, aiding them in reaching their innermost essence.

This framework leads us to the distinct stages of a Yoga Nidra script, each aligned with a specific Kosha. These stages form a sequence, guiding us deeper into the realm of the Self. In the subsequent sections, we'll explore these stages in greater detail.

Stages of Yoga Nidra & Koshas

Various traditions and contemporary forms of Yoga Nidra may have unique structures, yet they all share a common framework that generally encompasses the following stages. Here is the classical Satyananda Yoga Nidra© frame of a session, with some stages *italicized* to denote their absence in certain other schools of Yoga:

Relaxation
Sankalpa (first time): Setting a positive intention or resolution.
Rotation of Consciousness (body scan): Systematically directing awareness to different parts of the body.
Breath Awareness: Focusing on the breath and its rhythm.
Opposite Feelings: Exploring and integrating contrasting sensations.
Chidakasha: Observing the space of consciousness.
Visualisation: Guided mental imagery and journeys.
Sankalpa (second time): Reiterating the intention or resolution.
Closure: Gradually bringing awareness back to the physical surroundings.

Understanding the correspondences between these stages and the Koshas enriches your comprehension of the depth and purpose of each stage within a Yoga Nidra session.

Correspondences between Koshas & Yoga Nidra stages

Koshas	Stages of Yoga Nidra
Annamaya kosha	Preparation - Relaxation Rotation of Consciousness Closure
Pranayama kosha	Awareness of breath – Rotation of Consciousness
Manomaya kosha	Opposite senses Images, visualization
Vijnanamaya kosha	Chidakasha - Images, visualization
Anandamaya kosha	Chidakasha – although it is present in all of the stages and in the brief silence within the visualization.

This alignment helps the holistic integration of the physical, mental, and spiritual dimensions, guiding practitioners towards self-discovery and union.

Being aware of what impact each stage has will help you write more consistent Yoga Nidra scripts. So, we will now, see what are the effect and benefits of each stage.

INFLUENCE AND BENEFITS OF EACH STAGE

Preparation - Relaxation

Similar to a warm-up before physical exercise, the relaxation phase in Yoga Nidra serves as a mental and physical preparation. The practice of Yoga Nidra, conducted in the Savasana posture, challenges participants to let go and overcome resistance. By inducing relaxation, this stage readies the mind, body, and entire human system for the forthcoming Yoga Nidra practice. As participants reach a state of relaxation, they become more receptive and open to the rest of the session. Starting with relaxation sets the foundation for the entire practice, creating a sense of safety that fosters openness and willingness to be guided. All Yoga Nidra scripts should begin with relaxation. So always take five to ten minutes relaxing the body and mind.

Sankalpa

The second stage of a Yoga Nidra script introduces the participants to the concept of Sankalpa, or intention. Sankalpa is a positive statement that serves as the seed of transformation. It provides a clear and positive direction for the subconscious mind. The repetition of Sankalpa three times, infused with conviction, trust, and heightened sensory awareness, reinforces its impact.

Across all forms of Yoga Nidra, including Sankalpa, the commonality lies in its formulation: a concise, positive, and present-tense statement. It surpasses mere intention, operating as a resolute decision, an inducement directed toward the subconscious mind for fulfillment. Sankalpa thus acts as a potent tool for aligning one's conscious and subconscious aspirations, catalyzing positive change and growth.

Rotation of Consciousness

The rotation of consciousness is a technique that induces relaxation of the mind by relaxing the body. During this stage, participants are guided to focus their attention on various parts of the body.

In Satyananda Yoga Nidra©, the rotation of consciousness usually commences with the right hand thumb. In other variations of Yoga Nidra, the starting point can be the point between the eyebrows, and the Kundalini 61 points chart can be employed as a guide. The primary aim of this stage is to isolate the mind from external stimuli and sensory distractions. Participants are led through a comprehensive body scan. The scientific principle underlying this stage involves navigating sensations through the cerebral cortex, which, in turn, induces relaxation in the motor and sensory regions of the brain, thus benefiting both body and mind. The rotation of consciousness is conducted in two parts: awareness of specific body parts and awareness of the body as a whole.

Awareness of the Body (optional)

This phase delves deeper into the observer's state, fostering a connection with subtle senses. Participants remain grounded and entirely present. In Satyananda schools, individuals are often prompted to feel specific body parts and listen attentively – for instance, sensing the palms, feeling the lines, or noting the gentle contact of the lips. It's important to note that this stage may not be included in the scripts of many other Yoga Nidra forms.

Breath Awareness

Breath awareness enhances concentration and breathe management skills. It aids in the circulation of Prana (life force energy) and fortifies the mind. Through focused breathing, participants deepen the mental relaxation established during the rotation of consciousness, guiding them towards the stage of emotional relaxation. Breath awareness begins with a general observation of the breath – its flow and rhythm – and progresses to a deeper awareness of its qualities and sensations, fostering equilibrium and concentration. This stage often concludes with a countdown, contributing to heightened concentration and streamlining the mental processes. While the countdown is not mandatory, it serves as a remarkably effective deepening technique.

Opposite feelings (optional)

As we move into manomaya kosha, the mental body, we start to work with conceptual integration of sensation. The traditional form of Yoga Nidra Satyananda© uses pratipaksha bhavana, wherein participants experience opposite sensations and emotions.

Passing from one sensation (hot-cold) or emotion (happiness-sadness) to its opposite, creates balance. Here the participants realize, consciously or subconsciously, their ability to manage their feelings and reactions. It offers a chance to learn to control some subconscious functions. This stage aims to use associations to dissolve the conditional programming in our conscious and subconscious minds. It deepens the disconnection between the lower self and the higher self. It helps the practitioners to observe what with which they usually identify their selves and to understand that they are neither their emotions, nor their feelings or sensations. Moreover, through this stage they reinforce our inner power and will.

Chidakasha (optional)

Chidakasha, translated as the "space of consciousness," serves as the link between the conscious, subconscious, and superconscious realms. It is within this realm that mental phenomena manifest, appearing in various forms such as images, thoughts, and emotions. During this stage, practitioners focus on Chidakasha, observing the space and its contents, thus initiating the visualization process. For beginners, the exploration of Chidakasha may be omitted. This stage provides the mind with space and time to rest, enabling practitioners to distance themselves from their thoughts and connect with a higher dimension of themselves – the observer.

Participants are instructed to remain neutral observers, observing whatever arises behind their closed eyelids or forehead without criticism. It is crucial to prevent participants from slipping into a dream state or becoming carried away, ensuring they remain focused and attentive to your guidance. During the initial observation of Chidakasha, guide participants with care, as the nature of the experience is unpredictable. For some, the observation of a dark space might evoke anxiety, particularly in early sessions. Thus, especially during the initial stages, it's important to create an environment of safety and support.

It's worth noting that participants enter a vulnerable phase at this point, where their last defenses are left behind. Facilitate their sense of security and guide them to maintain a distance from Chidakasha, remaining observers rather than immersing themselves fully.

When integrated after visualization, the perception of Chidakasha becomes clearer and can serve as an opportunity for participants to connect with their higher selves, deepening their self-awareness and spiritual experience.

Visualization

During the visualization stage of Yoga Nidra, participants shift their awareness to the dark space in front of their closed eyes or the forehead, known as Chidakasha in yogic terminology. Visualization naturally follows this shift, as participants are guided to imagine specific symbols, images, situations, or narratives. This stage is akin to embarking on a journey within a journey.

In this phase, participants experience the interplay between their outer and inner worlds. Through visualization, they may encounter unconscious imprints, gain insight into their triggers, and cultivate a greater sense of control over their mental and emotional responses. The relaxed mind responds to the practice with deep-rooted cleansing, possibly leading to the liberation of memories and the creation of new neural pathways in the brain.

Coming Back

After guiding participants through the visualization journey, it is crucial to facilitate their return to waking consciousness. This transition should be as gentle and gradual as the initial induction. If you introduced a Sankalpa at the beginning, this is an opportune moment to remind participants of their resolution and ask them to repeat it once more.

Incorporating layers of identifying joy, well-being, and bliss, as seen in iRest© Yoga Nidra, aids students in connecting with gratitude and presence, enhancing their overall experience. Guide participants by gradually shifting their attention back to their breath, body, and the physical space around them, effectively moving from inner to outer awareness.

Once the return is complete, encourage participants to slowly move their bodies and stretch, allowing them to adjust to the transition. As a trainer, remember that just as a deep dive necessitates careful ascent, the return from the depths of Yoga Nidra should be gradual to prevent abrupt shifts in mental and physical states. Offer ample time for the mind and body to recalibrate.

Closing

Towards the end of the session, following the same order used at the beginning—breath, sense of the body, sense of space, outward senses, and bodily movements—provides a sense of symmetry and closure.

Bringing the listener back to a state of complete relaxation before they open their eyes is a skillful way to conclude the guided meditation. Techniques that were used to induce relaxation initially can be employed to guide the listener back to a state of awareness. Alternatively, uplifting phrases or calming affirmations, such as "I am at peace," "I am relaxed," or "I am healed," can be repeated to aid in the transition.

Finally, wrap up the meditation by summarizing the key elements covered during the session and expressing gratitude. This closure allows participants to leave the practice feeling centered, refreshed, and connected.

WRITING YOUR OWN SCRIPT FROM SCRATCH

Preparation - Relaxation

The process of achieving general relaxation can be approached in various ways. You will find below, different techniques that can be combined:

- Start by directing the listener's focus towards their breath, inviting them to notice the gentle rise and fall of their chest and belly with each breath.
- Assist them in releasing any tension held in their body through a quick body scan, acknowledging areas of tension and letting them go. You might choose to emphasize the points of contact between the body and the ground. Alternatively, guide practitioners to gently tense and release muscles or recall a pleasant memory to induce a sense of well-being.
- Consider initiating the relaxation either from the feet to enhance grounding or from the head to facilitate detachment from thoughts.
- Encourage the participants to recollect a positive moment from their day or life. This evokes a feeling of

joy and helps them disconnect from current worries, utilizing the brain's ability to blend imagination and reality.

- Pose a question such as, "Imagine how deeply relaxed you could feel throughout this session?" to stimulate imagination and facilitate inner tranquility.
- Counting breaths for a brief period is an effective tension-release technique. While countdowns can be employed at various stages, in Yoga Nidra scripts, it might work best during the breath awareness phase as a deepener.

- Capture their imagination with a brief visualization, such as imagining their thoughts being written on paper and placed in a drawer, or feeling a warm breeze gently caressing their body, creating a sense of ideal temperature. Describe relaxing scenes, such as the body melting like butter.
- In the classical Satyananda Yoga Nidra© tradition, the Antar Mouna technique focuses on sounds. You can begin by asking participants to focus on distant sounds and gradually bring the attention closer, or simply start by acknowledging all sounds, then the silence between them, immersing oneself in that silence.

The primary objective is to establish a sense of safety initially, enabling practitioners to release tension. Then, guide their attention from external to internal, promoting grounding for sustained awareness throughout the session. Ensuring participants are fully present in the here and now is essential.

A word of caution: This stage is crucial, as relaxation lays the foundation for further self-exploration. Approach it with kindness and sensitivity. Tailor the process to each participant's needs to cultivate a sense of safety and encourage maximum relaxation.

Sankalpa (optional)

Swami Satyananda popularized the concept of Sankalpa in Yoga Nidra, although in the traditional Indian yoga tradition, the ultimate goal is to transcend all desires. While the exact reasons are not clear, it is presumed that this concept may have roots in the Tantric tradition of setting intentions.

- In certain variations of Yoga Nidra, the intention may pertain solely to the practice itself. For example, one might set intentions like "I will maintain awareness throughout the entire session" or "I am present and at ease in this moment."
- In other instances, the practitioner is guided to adopt a specific Sankalpa. The instructor presents a universal intention, such as courage, love, inner peace, or fulfillment, for all participants.
- Alternatively, the intention can stem from a personal goal or desire. It signifies an inner state the practitioner aspires to manifest in their life.
- Some forms of Yoga Nidra omit the use of Sankalpa altogether.

What remains consistent across all forms of Yoga Nidra, including Sankalpa, is that it is conveyed through a concise, positive statement, framed in the present tense. It transcends mere intention; for some, it becomes a decision, while for others, an instruction delivered to the subconscious mind for realization. In its more spiritual manifestation, Sankalpa is an inspiration that emerges naturally, rather than being consciously formulated.

When allowing participants to craft their own Sankalpa, it is vital to provide clear guidance on the creation process. These instructions can be given at this stage, before the beginning of the session, or both. Emphasize that the Sankalpa should be personal, devoid of external references, and phrased as if it has already been achieved. In my personal opinion, avoiding phrases like "I want,"

"I believe," or "I imagine" can be quite effective, although certain schools may use them.

Additionally, the Sankalpa must be positive and not imply a negative circumstance. For instance, using "cure" assumes an ailment. In this context, it's preferable for participants to state "I am strong, I am healthy." While there are no strict rules, some schools might employ Sankalpa with negative phrasing, such as "I do not smoke." Personally, as a Life Coach with NLP expertise and considering the latest scientific insights, I am inclined to believe that this is not the optimal way to communicate with the subconscious mind.

A word of caution: Certain beliefs and values could conflict with the concept of Sankalpa, leading participants to experience resistance. Often, this resistance is rooted in unconscious beliefs or values. Whenever possible, assist these participants in formulating a Sankalpa that the subconscious mind can embrace as attainable.
Above all, the crucial aspect is that the decision should be imprinted with unwavering determination and aligned emotions.

Rotation of Awareness

Initiating the rotation of awareness may appear intuitive to commence with the right side, yet there are no fixed rules. Notably, the Satyananda approach begins at the right thumb, while the Himalaya method begins at the crown of the head. Some practitioners opt to focus solely on major body segments (front, back, top, and bottom) or exclusively on joints. Others opt to direct their attention toward the chakra centers.

- Encourage participants to concentrate on each part as you mention them.
- Alternatively, you can prompt participants to mentally repeat the names of the body parts after you. This technique greatly assists beginners in maintaining concentration, active participation,

preventing boredom, and sustaining alertness, thus minimizing the likelihood of drifting into sleep.
- Or guide them to vividly visualize each part of the body.
- As participants gain more experience, you can incorporate additional visualizations, like envisioning a beam of light, a droplet of water, or the sensations of warmth or coolness.
- For novice learners, it is advisable to focus solely on external body regions. After ample practice, consider introducing joints, followed by organs. Eventually, progress to exploring the various chakra centers, transitioning from the physical realm to the realm of energy.

Second Part – Concluding the Rotation of Awareness (optional)
The conclusion involves deliberate shifts in awareness:

- from toes to head or head to toes
- from back to front
- from left to right
- from upper body to lower body
- from limbs to head to torso

Continuing until the point where awareness envelops the entirety of the body.

Word of Caution: *There exists no definitive methodology, except that while guiding consciousness through the physical body, it is crucial to ensure participants consciously traverse each point. When working with individuals grappling with chronic pain, it might be necessary to omit certain body parts, especially when addressing specific areas of discomfort.*
It is important to keep in mind that as a facilitator, your approach can be adapted to the unique needs and circumstances of your participants. Flexibility and attentiveness are key to ensuring a comfortable and effective experience during the rotation of awareness practice.

Some samples of rotation of awareness

<u>Short Version:</u>

Right heel. Left heel. Right calf. Left calf. Right knee. Left knee. Right thigh. Left thigh. Right hip. Left hip. Both hips together. Lower back. Belly. Middle back. Stomach. Upper back. Torso. Right hand. Left hand. Right wrist. Left wrist. Right forearm. Left forearm. Right elbow. Left elbow. Right upper arm. Left upper arm. Right shoulder. Left shoulder. Both shoulders together. Neck. Throat. Back of head. Face. All points of contact with the earth…

<u>Long Version:</u>

Direct your attention to the right hand. Begin with the right hand thumb. Move to the second finger. Proceed to the third finger. Shift to the fourth finger. Finally, focus on the little finger. Transition to the palm of the hand. Now, move to the back of the hand. Continue to the wrist. Proceed along the forearm. Shift your awareness to the elbow. Gradually move up to the upper arm.

Direct your attention to the shoulder. Now, shift to the right armpit. Move to the ribs on the right side. Then, the waist. Continue down to the right hip. Proceed to the right thigh. Shift your focus to the knee. Move down to the calf. Gradually reach the ankle. Direct your awareness to the heel. Move along to the sole of the foot. Then, transition to the top of the foot. Finally, shift your attention to the right big toe. Proceed to the second toe. Move to the third toe. Shift to the fourth toe. Finally, focus on the little toe.

Now, shift your focus to the left hand. Begin with the left hand thumb. Move to the second finger. Proceed to the third finger. Shift to the fourth finger. Finally, focus on the little finger. Transition to the palm of the hand. Now, move to the back of the hand. Continue to the wrist. Proceed along the forearm. Shift your awareness to the elbow. Gradually move up to the upper arm. Direct your attention to the shoulder. Now, shift to the left armpit. Move to the ribs on the left side. Then, the waist. Continue down to the left hip. Proceed to the left thigh. Shift your focus to the knee. Move down to the calf. Gradually reach the ankle. Direct your awareness to the heel. Move along to the sole of the foot. Then, transition to the top of the foot. Finally, shift your attention to the left big toe. Proceed to the second toe. Move to the third toe. Shift to the fourth toe. Finally, focus on the little toe.

Continue to the top of the head. Move to the forehead. Proceed to both temples. Shift to the right eyebrow. Move to the left eyebrow. Focus on the space between the eyebrows. Shift to the right eyelid. Move to the left eyelid. Direct your attention to the right eye. Move to the left eye. Shift your focus to the right ear. Move to the left ear. Proceed to the right inner ear. Shift to the left inner ear. Now, bring your awareness to both cheeks. Move on to the nose. Shift your focus to the tip of the nose. Move to the right nostril. Proceed to the left nostril.

Shift your attention to the upper lip. Move to the lower lip. Now, focus on the jaws. Transition your awareness to your mouth. Become aware of your tongue, teeth, gums, and roof of the mouth. Now, shift to your chin. Proceed to the throat. Move to the right collar bone. Shift to the left collar bone. Focus on the right chest. Move to the left chest. Now, direct your attention to the middle chest. Shift to the upper abdomen. Move to the navel. Proceed to the lower abdomen. Shift your focus to the groin.

From the groin, shift to the right buttock. Move to the left buttock. Focus on the lower back. Move to the mid-back. Shift to the upper back. Now, direct your attention to the right shoulder blade. Proceed to the left shoulder blade. Shift your focus to the neck. Move to the back of the head. Now, encompass the entire spine. Gradually expand your awareness to cover the whole head. Shift to the right arm. Move to the left arm. Now, focus on both arms together. Shift to the whole right leg. Proceed to the whole left leg.

Finally, encompass both legs together. Now, bring your awareness to the entire front body. Gradually shift your focus to the entire back body. Finally, be fully aware of your entire body.

Remember, there is no fixed way to do this practice, and you can adjust the sequence based on your preferences and the needs of your participants.

<u>**61 points version**</u>

1. Point between the eyebrows
2. Center of the throat
3. Right shoulder joint
4. Right elbow joint
5. Middle of the right wrist
6. Tip of the right thumb
7. Tip of the index finger
8. Tip of the middle finger
9. Tip of the fourth finger (ring finger)
10. Tip of the small finger
11. Right wrist joint
12. Right elbow joint
13. Right shoulder joint
14. Center of the throat

15. Left shoulder joint
16. Left elbow joint
17. Middle of the left wrist
18. Tip of the left thumb
19. Tip of the index finger
20. Tip of the middle finger
21. Tip of the fourth finger (ring finger)
22. Tip of the small finger
23. Left wrist joint
24. Left elbow joint
25. Left shoulder joint
26. Center of the throat

27. Heart center
28. Right nipple
29. Heart center
30. Left nipple
31. Heart center

32. Solar plexus

33.   Navel center (2 inches below the physical navel)
34.   Right hip joint
35.   Right knee joint
36.   Right ankle joint
37.   Right big toe
38.   Tip of the second toe
39.   Tip of the third toe
40.   Tip of the fourth toe
41.   Tip of the small toe
42.   Right ankle joint
43.   Right knee joint
44.   Right hip joint
45.   Navel center (2 inches below physical navel)

46.   Left hip joint
47.   Left knee joint
48.   Left ankle joint
49.   Left big toe
50.   Tip of the second toe
51.   Tip of the third toe
52.   Tip of the fourth toe
53.   Tip of the small toe
54.   Left ankle joint
55.   Left knee joint
56.   Left hip joint
57.   Navel center (2 inches below physical navel)

58.   Solar plexus
59.   Heart center
60.   Center of the throat
61.   Center between the eyebrows

Word of Caution: *In this practice, your aim is to guide participants into a state of deep bodily awareness, encouraging them to genuinely sense each part as it is mentioned. To effectively achieve this,* *consider instructing participants to silently echo the name of each body part after you. This technique is instrumental in anchoring their presence in the present moment, preventing their attention from wandering elsewhere. The cornerstone of success lies in maintaining an appropriate pace.*

To determine the optimal pace, mentally rehearse each body part as you name them aloud. This seamless continuity ensures a smooth progression, leaving no room for attention to drift away. Remember, the rhythm you establish plays a pivotal role in engaging participants and fostering an immersive experience.

Awareness of the Body (optional)

During this phase, participants delve deeper into the observer's state, attuning themselves to their most subtle senses. This stage serves to ensure their grounding while maintaining full presence. Typically, participants are guided to meticulously feel specific, delicate areas of the body. Examples include gently sensing the lines on the palms, the subtle point of contact of the lips, or the delicate touch of the eyelids.

Breath Awareness

This section of the practice offers a fluidity that accommodates various approaches. Whether you opt for breathing techniques, breath counting, visualization of the breath, or any other method, the primary objective remains cultivating a profound connection with the breath.

Initially, participants are encouraged to witness the breath without attempting to alter it. From this foundational step, a range of practices can be introduced, such as:

- Counting the breath using multiples of 108. For instance, counting backward from 54 to 1 or from 27 to 1.

- Engaging participants in mental breathing techniques like:

Dirgha: Introducing participants to yogic breathing, enabling them to guide their breath for maximum expansion.

Ujjayi Pranayama: Enhancing concentration through regulated breathing.

Nadi Shodhana or Anuloma Viloma: Visualizing and sensing breath flow through alternate nostrils, experiencing the union of the two flows at the end of the inhale and their separation at the beginning of the exhale.

Brahmari: Encouraging participants to listen to the sound of their breath within their minds or feel the sound resonating in different body parts.

Sama Vritti: Equalized breath at 4 or 5 counts.

4-count Inhale/8-counts Exhale Ratio: Guiding participants through a specific breath rhythm.

*A **word of caution**: When introducing pranayama techniques, it's prudent to do so gradually. Some participants may not have encountered breathwork of this nature before and may require guidance. Allocate a few minutes at the start of the session to introduce and guide participants through the specific pranayama technique you intend to incorporate. This foundational instruction will ensure a cohesive and effective experience as they proceed with the practice.*

Opposite Feelings (optional)

Exercise caution regarding the length of descriptions in this phase. The body's inherent quest for equilibrium naturally generates opposing sensations. When descriptions are overly brief, participants might not have ample time to cultivate these sensations. Conversely, overly extensive descriptions can prompt the body to generate the opposing sensation prematurely. To enhance the exploration of sensations, invite participants to recollect moments from their past when they experienced specific feelings (e.g., cold, heavy, warm, light).

- Sensations can encompass physical, mental, or emotional dimensions.
- Visualization can also be used, describing scenarios where participants would experience these sensations. For instance, describe a scenario of being barefoot in a frigid winter wind.
- Employ sensations and feelings that are complementary opposites. Do not propose cold and wet but cold and warm or wet and dry.
- Leverage the breath, particularly for sensations of heaviness and lightness. Inhale for lightness, exhale for heaviness.
- Begin with the negative emotion or sensation and shift to the positive one, preserving an overall pleasant inner state.
- Do one pair of opposite sensation after another (e.g., cold-hot and heavy-light).
- With practice, participants can transition back and forth between opposing states, striving to reach the middle ground where neither extreme exists.
- Integrating opposite feelings into visualizations can also be effective.

Word of Caution: *Keep in mind that certain sensations might trigger negative experiences for some participants. For instance, survivors of domestic violence or those in eating disorder recovery could be sensitive to sensations of heaviness and lightness. Choose language thoughtfully and always encourage participants to return to the awareness of breath if any discomfort arises.*

Chidakasha

Chidakasha is often described as an infinite expanse of darkness, reminiscent of deep blue velvet. The description you employ for Chidakasha can profoundly influence the practitioner's sense of security. Thus, incorporating key words that evoke safety, such as "warm," "safe," and "friendly," is advisable.

Consider Chidakasha as analogous to your mind, with distinct layers including the conscious, subconscious, and hyperconscious aspects. Just as in the broader Yoga Nidra practice, progression should unfold from the more tangible to the subtle realms.

Various metaphors can illustrate Chidakasha:

- A sea, a night of new moon, with no stars in the in the sky.
- A dimly lit room with a screen stands on the front wall, projecting visions and on the floor or back wall, a small opening or door beckons exploration.
- A theater with its entrance, seating area, stage where phenomena manifest, and backstage. And a secondary door which might be found backstage, leading toward the Higher Self.
- A cinema complete with its screen.
- A cave...

Word of Caution: *For beginners, advise a degree of detachment while observing Chidakasha. Encourage them to observe from a distance rather than becoming immersed. The general principle is to prevent participants from becoming disconnected in a "no-man's-land" and to maintain ongoing awareness of their experiences throughout the practice.*

Visualization

Once the participant's awareness is focused, we guide them to engage in visualization by using symbols, images, or initiating a mental journey. The challenge lies in maintaining their focus and preventing them from drifting off into daydreams or creating their own visualizations. While some may argue that controlling this is beyond our reach, I firmly believe that the teacher and their script bear 50% of the responsibility.

It's crucial to strike a balance with your script – neither too lengthy nor too concise. It should provide adequate details while also allowing room for participants to fill in from their own imagination. The pacing should neither be too fast nor too slow. Yes, I hear you... This is where experience becomes invaluable. Don't worry; you'll get the hang of it. I'm confident.

Two primary types of visualization exist: the list of symbols or images and the narrative approach or story.

List of symbols or images:
The list of symbols or images serves as an excellent starting point for beginners. It aids in the development of their visualization skills, teaching them how to recreate symbols and images using all their senses. This approach is also safer, as it carries a lower risk of triggering negative emotions. The symbols or images should be named relatively quickly, preventing participants from dwelling or overthinking. Repeat the name of each symbol or image rhythmically three times before transitioning to the next.

- Initially, aim for simplicity, avoiding excessive detail. For instance: candle, mountain, crow, house, chimney...
- Over time, progress to more intricate symbols or images. For example: a burning candle, a snow-covered mountain, a flying crow...
- Eventually, encourage participants to incorporate their senses. For instance: a warm cup of tea, the scent of

burning incense, the taste of lemon...

- Symbols or images can contrast, encompassing both positive and negative aspects. Some of those are: a bright sun and purring rain, a confined space and an expansive area. These opposite representations neutralize each other but engage the brain's left hemisphere. This practice diminishes the polarization of our perceptions concerning good and bad, right and wrong.

A word of caution: Certain images or scenarios may trigger memories, impressions, or emotions. Each image evokes something unique for every individual, based on their life experiences. The challenge lies in the unpredictability of what an image or scenario might evoke. Therefore, exercise caution when selecting images and scenarios, and always conclude with a positive one.

Stories

Visualizations using a story are best fit for people having some experience than for beginners. Due to its complexity, maintaining focus can prove challenging. Novices might easily become engrossed in crafting their own narrative instead of adhering to your guidance.

That being said, a story is essentially a collection of interconnected scenes (images) united by an overarching, desired outcome—the ultimate destination of your journey.

Determining the Ultimate Destination:

The first step in writing a Yoga Nidra visualization script is to pinpoint the lesson, experience, or growth you wish participants to attain. Visualization stories mirror journeys; the central theme or intended outcome serves as your ultimate destination. Here are several potential desired outcomes to consider:

- Self-confidence
- Self-esteem
- Fulfillment

- Self-love and self-acceptance
- Release
- Cultivation of gratitude
- Concepts like truth, compassion, and tolerance

Once you have selected the desired outcome for your story, you will have established where you intend to lead your participants. However, you must still determine the route—the path—you'll take to get them there.

Choosing the Path:

Life is a mixture of highs and lows, challenges and ease. The path parallels those various life moments, encompassing achievements, setbacks, and healing.
To chart the path leading to your intended destination, consider these questions:

- How does one attain this inner state?
- What real-life factors contribute to the development of these attributes?
- What life experiences shape a person who embodies these strengths?

Strive to avoid triggering intense negative emotions, while also integrating some challenges that mirror life's complexities. However, select challenges judiciously to avoid overwhelming participants.
Imagine challenges that participants can manage successfully. These challenges might involve overcoming fear, anxiety, sadness, or stress. For instance, if your story involves climbing a mountain, you might introduce a segment where the path becomes arduous, invoking sensations of fatigue, describing a burdensome backpack, or illustrating unfavorable weather conditions.

To identify appropriate challenges, consider these steps:

- Begin with your intended destination—the desired outcome—and determine the opposite emotion or feeling. Example: Low self-confidence stands in opposition to self-confidence, with doubt and fear accompanying the former.
- Delve into the feelings of an individual lacking self-confidence.
- Visualize their typical reactions in various life situations.
- Identify triggers for diminished self-confidence.

Use your own experiences to enhance the narrative's impact.

With the departure point, ultimate destination, and chosen path established, it's time to craft the narrative content. Adhering to the structure outlined below will be invaluable.

Structure of the Story:

Creating a visualization story is like writing any story; it involves a beginning (departure point), progression (the path - the story's climax), and conclusion (arrival point). The following structured points offer guidance to shape your story.

Here are some tips:

1. **Establish the Setting – Departure Point:** Describe the environment, the context, the companions, and the timeframe. Paint a vivid picture of where, with whom, and when the story begins.

Question – where, who, and when?

2. **Initiate an Action:** Introduce an action or activity that engages the participants, giving momentum to the story.

Question - what they are doing?

3. **Convey Emotions:** Describe the emotions experienced by the characters, helping participants connect with their feelings.

Question - how do they feel?

4. **Present Obstacles:** Introduce challenges that align with real-life obstacles your metaphor addresses. These obstacles serve as triggers for the emotions you aim to address. Examples could be facing a closed door or climbing a high mountain.

Question – what makes it difficult to achieve?

5. **Provide Resources:** Offer participants resources to surmount the obstacles. These resources should correspond to the desired real-life outcome of the metaphor. Resources can be imaginary or realistic, like discovering a key under a vase or receiving assistance from a helpful figure.

Question – What is the best resource? What would help in such situation?

6. **Achieve the Outcome:** Guide participants to successfully attain the desired emotional state or outcome. Regardless of the situation or emotions, emphasize their achievement and success.

Question – What is the desired outcome?

7. **Acknowledge Emotions:** Allow participants time to acknowledge their emotions, either by describing them or simply feeling them.

Question – How will they feel when attaining the desired outcome?

8. **Absorb Knowledge:** Encourage participants to absorb the lessons learned from the experience. Ask them to identify where they feel the positive emotion, its shape, color, and significance.

Once the structure of your story is in place, it's time to populate each section with images or scenes.

The Power of Metaphors:

Yoga Nidra visualization scripts employ metaphors, which are symbolic stories conveying a message that can lead to positive transformations in attitudes, beliefs, and lives. Metaphors engage without triggering critical thinking, reducing resistance. The power of metaphors is their ability to address a theme indirectly, capturing its essence.

Each segment of your story represents a step toward the intended positive emotional experience. This is why metaphors should stem from genuine life experiences. For instance, guiding participants to ascend a mountain reflects the theme of self-confidence through goal attainment. Other scenes may introduce fantastical elements like flying above the body (theme: recognizing one's identity beyond the physical).

Given participants' diverse life experiences, you cannot predict how metaphors will resonate. For example: water can be a negative trigger for someone who experienced drowning.

Therefore, provide a safety tool to prevent potent negative emotions. For example:

- For water-related fears: Offer the ability to breathe underwater or emerge at will.
- For fear of darkness: Provide a flashlight.

Symbolism Ideas:

- Mountains symbolize challenges, with their height representing difficulty levels. Hills present milder challenges.
- Rivers signify an unceasing flow of time, unstoppable like the current.
- Weeds represent invasive thoughts or feelings, crowding out positive elements.
- Sun symbolizes warmth, brightness, and life, shining on all unconditionally. It is the source of all life. It shines during the day and at night reflect on the moon,

it is the conscious part of the mind, masculine and active energy.

- Moon is a cold, enigmatic light that illuminates the darkness, representing the subconscious. The moon reflects the light of the sun in the dark. It represents the subconscious part of the mind, feminine and passive energy.
- Forests mirror the subconscious mind, with trees and plants symbolizing thoughts. Paths within represent choices.
- Caves mirror the subconscious, offering protection and isolation within the forest of thoughts.

A world of caution: Describe images or narrate at a steady pace, neither too rapid nor too sluggish. This allows participants to stay in their subconscious realm. Since the subconscious operates faster than the conscious, maintaining a steady pace ensures participants can grasp and analyze the information comfortably.

Conclusion and Transitioning Back:

As I have emphasized throughout, your visualization script parallels a journey, akin to any other narrative. Concluding it thoughtfully is important. You aim for participants to retain the positive emotions, feelings, and strengths they have experienced, being able to integrate them into their daily lives seamlessly.

Abruptly ending the script could undermine the progress achieved thus far. To ensure a smooth transition back, consider employing the following approaches:

1. Dissolving Imagery: Tell participants that the imagery they have experienced is now dissolving, much like a cloud in the sky. Emphasize that what remains are the newfound positive emotions, sensations, and strengths.
2. Guided Return: Lead participants back to the point where the visualization began. If it was in front of a forest, guide them swiftly out of the forest and then

allow the mental picture to fade away.

3. Chidakasha Return: If your visualization initiated with Chidakasha, gently guide participants back by having them focus on the infinite, welcoming darkness of Chidakasha.

Consider concluding the practice with a positive affirmation that reinforces the experience and the impact of the practice. For instance, "I am at peace with myself and the world around me."

Armed with these insights, you are well-equipped to craft a compelling visualization story. To further enhance the potency of your narrative, delve into the upcoming chapter, where you will find additional tips for maximizing the impact of your story.

ENHANCING YOUR VISUALISATION SCRIPT

1. **Use Clear and Concise Language**: Recognize the significant impact of language and imagery on the practitioner's experience. Use clear language, avoiding confusion or intricacy in your instructions to ensure participants can easily follow your instructions. Avoid complex vocabulary that might engage the conscious mind and disrupt the desired state of surrender. Tailor your imagery to align with the intended purpose of the practice.

2. **Sensory Engagement**: Give the participants a chance to use all of their senses. Involve all senses by incorporating sensory cues like visual descriptions, sounds, and scents. This enhances participant's immersion and amplifies the vividness of their experience. Utilizing sensory language makes it easier for the picture to appear in their mind and deepens their sense of inner awareness.

3. **Use action-oriented verbs**: Employ action-oriented verbs to encourage engagement. Prompt participants to "walk," "listen,"

"feel," "observe," and "experience." This draws them into the experience and fosters a deeper connection.
Some phrases you could use are:

Watch the environment instead of describing it so they can let their subconscious fill the blank.
Listen to the birds
Take the book from the shelf.
Smell flowers.

4. **Incorporate Questions**: Pose questions that prompt participants to engage with their environment and sensations. For instance, inquire about how their body feels, the color of the sky, the size of objects, the weather, or any audible sounds. This fosters a deeper sense of inner awareness.
Examples of questions are:

How do your body feel?
What color is the sky?
What size is the door?
What is the weather?
Is there some sounds?

5. **Immersive Language**: Use descriptive language to facilitate immersion. Encourage participants to visualize by saying "imagine" or "picture," allowing their subconscious to paint the scene. For example, "Imagine walking through a lush forest with towering trees..."

6. **Use the verb "may"** will bring their attention where you want it to be without them feeling pressured and obliged to succeed. E.g.: you may feel the grass under your feet, you may hear some voices far away, you may....

7. **Select the Details**: Prioritize relevant details in your description. Highlight elements that contribute to the intended

experience, while omitting superfluous details. For instance, if the type of trees isn't integral to the story, there's no need to elaborate on them.

8. **Avoid negative forms**: Do not use "not". You will not feel scared will surely make the participants thing about fear. The right formula is "you feel safe".

9. **Pause and Silence**: Offer moments of silence to allow participants to fully absorb their surroundings and sensations. These pauses encourage a sense of presence and mindfulness.

10. **Use Affirmations** when it comes to the arrival point. Here you do not suggest how they may feel but rather tell them. For instance, "You are feeling fulfilled, relaxed.", "see how it is for you to feel fulfilled, relaxed.", or "listen to the tone of your inner voice when you are fulfilled, relaxed."

11. **Emphasize Safety & Relaxation** reminding them regularly that they are safe and secured. Give them a tool that they can use in case they do not feel well. It could be a phone, a torch, a friend… Taking the above example where they walk a path in a forest you may say that the sun makes the forest to be bright and shiny or tell them that whenever they want they can come back to where they began… Emphasize the importance of relaxation throughout the practice. Encourage the listener to release any tension or stress and allow themselves to fully relax and let go.

12. **Be Flexible**: While maintaining structure, allow room for personal interpretation. Leave aspects open-ended, enabling participants to fill in details with their own experiences and imagination.

13. **Script size**: Your script should not be too long. If you spend too much time describing specifics, it may sound over complicated. In any case, it's a good idea to give the listener the opportunity to

expand upon your suggested visualizations.

14. **Give space to Personal Experience**: especially when it comes to the arrival point. Do not suggest how they should feel. Instead, name the feeling but avoid describing it. Let them create experience it in any way they want. Example: You are feeling fulfilled, relaxed... see how it is for you to feel fulfilled, relaxed... listen to the tone of your inner voice when you are fulfilled, relaxed...

15. **End with a Positive Reinforcement**: Integrate positive affirmations or reinforcing statements throughout the script to enhance the intended outcome. These affirmations contribute to the overall impact of the experience.
Ending with a positive statement will help the participants carry the positive emotion, feeling or strength they experienced during the practice into their daily life.

By using these tips, you will create a rich and immersive visualization that resonates deeply with participants, facilitating a transformative journey and ensuring a fulfilling conclusion to your Yoga Nidra practice.

THINGS TO CONSIDER FOR THE WHOLE SESSION

Holistic Approach: Recognize the interconnectedness of each stage in your Yoga Nidra session. Every phase contributes to the next, propelling participants toward the final goal of fulfillment and joy. Ensure that each step is meticulously planned and seamlessly connected to the others, maintaining a coherent and fluid progression. Remember the aim is to move from the outer to the inner, from the gross to the subtle.

Maintain the Ultimate Purpose: While choosing a desired outcome is crucial, always hold in mind the overarching purpose of Yoga Nidra: to unite with the True Self. This awareness will infuse your scripts with profound significance and empower participants, regardless of their circumstances, as they journey towards self-realization.

Adaptability for Diverse Audiences: Yoga Nidra scripts are versatile and can be tailored to diverse audiences and objectives. Adjust scripts to cater to children, seniors, or individuals with specific health considerations. Modify language, imagery, and techniques to suit the unique needs and capabilities of your target audience.

Varied Purposes: Acknowledge the potential applications of Yoga Nidra, ranging from stress alleviation and improved sleep to spiritual growth. Tailor your scripts to serve specific objectives, ensuring that the language and content align with the intended purpose.

Transitions and Flow: Pay special attention to smooth transitions between different stages of the session. Seamless flow enhances the participants' immersion and maintains their engagement.

Universal Themes: Integrate universal themes that resonate across various backgrounds and cultures, fostering a relatable experience for participants from diverse walks of life.

Empowerment and Fulfillment: Infuse your script with empowering language and affirmations that reinforce the journey towards self-discovery and fulfillment.

Intentional Language: Be intentional with the language you choose, ensuring it aligns with the overarching purpose and desired outcome of the practice. Each word should contribute to the intended impact.

Evolving Scripts: Regularly revisit and revise your scripts to incorporate new insights, techniques, and experiences. This allows your scripts to evolve and remain relevant over time.

By considering these factors, you can craft a comprehensive Yoga Nidra session that guides participants on a transformative journey, nurturing their connection with the True Self and fostering a sense of profound fulfillment.

REVIEW & REFINE YOUR SCRIPTS

1. **Self-Testing**: Once your Yoga Nidra script is written, it's vital to test it yourself. Read it aloud or record your voice reading it, then listen to it as if you were a participant. This process helps you evaluate the script's effectiveness and identify areas for improvement.
2. **Optimal Length**: While testing, note sections where the script appears too lengthy or excessively concise. Strive to retain only the most essential words and phrases, maintaining a balanced pacing throughout the session.
3. **Imagery Alignment**: Pay attention to the coherence between your envisioned experience and the imagery your script guides participants to imagine. Ensuring alignment between these two elements fosters a more immersive and congruent experience.
4. **Pauses**: Observe where pauses or moments of reflection should be inserted. These pauses allow participants to engage fully in the experience and internalize the journey. Make note of the timings for these pauses to maintain a harmonious pace.
5. **Language Consistency**: Ensure the language used in the script aligns seamlessly with the imaginative

experience. Consistency in language enhances participants' ability to connect with the visualization.

6. **Participants Engagement**: Consider where you can enhance engagement and immersion for participants. Identify moments where the script can encourage participants to explore sensations, emotions, or imagery more deeply.

7. **Narrative Flow**: Evaluate the overall flow of the script. Verify that each stage leads naturally into the next, creating a coherent and captivating narrative.

8. **Adaptable Script**: Assess if the script can be adapted for different audiences or purposes. Make any necessary modifications to ensure flexibility and relevance for various participants and objectives.

9. **Refinement and Improvement**: Identify aspects of the script that could benefit from refinement. Make necessary revisions to enhance clarity, effectiveness, and alignment with your intended outcomes.

10. **Trial and Iteration**: After making improvements, conduct additional self-testing and refinement as needed. Iterate through this process until you're satisfied with the script's quality and impact.

11. **Peer Feedback**: Consider seeking feedback from peers or colleagues experienced in Yoga Nidra or guided visualization practices. Their insights can provide valuable perspectives and help further refine your script.

By rigorously self-testing and refining your scripts, you ensure that they deliver a compelling and transformative experience for participants, guiding them on a meaningful journey of self-discovery and realization.

TEACHING YOGA NIDRA

Leading a Yoga Nidra Session
Leading a Yoga Nidra session involves more than merely reading a script. It requires skillful guidance and the ability to create a safe and conducive environment for deep relaxation. Techniques for leading a session include setting an intention, pacing the script effectively, using a calm and soothing tone of voice, and providing gentle reminders to stay present and relaxed.

Creating a Comfortable Environment
Ensure that the space is comfortable, quiet, and free from distractions. Soft lighting, calming music, or no music at all, and props such as blankets and bolsters will help build a safe and relaxing atmosphere.

Dos and Don'ts of Leading Yoga Nidra
Find the right pace for each stage. Speak clearly, use inclusive language, and provide clear instructions. Avoid interrupting the participants' experience and making assumptions about their experience.

Language and Tone
Language and tone differ among the various schools of Yoga. Some give instructions in a monotone way and with authority.

Others use a more calming, soothing, and supportive tone. What matters is that your tone reflects the confidence you feel about guiding the participants during their journey.

SUMMARY OF
KEY POINTS

- ✓ Yoga Nidra is a powerful relaxation and meditation practice that can help reduce stress, improve sleep, and promote overall well-being.
- ✓ Writing an effective Yoga Nidra script involves setting clear intentions, using language and imagery effectively, incorporating relaxation techniques, and creating a positive and safe environment.
- ✓ Leading a Yoga Nidra session requires skillful guidance, including setting an intention, pacing the script effectively, using the right tone of voice, and providing gentle reminders to stay present and relaxed.
- ✓ Yoga Nidra sessions can be adapted to meet the needs of different audiences and serve different purposes.
- ✓ Practicing Yoga Nidra regularly can lead to numerous benefits, including improved sleep, reduced stress and anxiety, and enhanced overall well-being.
- ✓ Additional resources such as books, websites, and workshops can provide you further guidance and support.

Overall, the key point to emphasize is the importance of effective script writing and skillful guidance in leading Yoga Nidra sessions to help practitioners experience the full benefits of this powerful practice.

FINAL THOUGHTS

"Congratulations, dear reader, on completing this comprehensive guide to write a remarkable Yoga Nidra script!
You possess now the invaluable tools to create transformative experiences for yourself and others.

Embrace your creativity as you design your Yoga Nidra scripts. Trust the process, allowing your words to flow from your heart and mind.
Tailor your scripts to the unique needs and intentions of your audience, acknowledging their individual journeys and aspirations.
Lastly, as you share your creations, remember that your presence and intention are just as important as the words you speak.
Cultivate a nurturing environment, free from judgment and expectation, where your participants can surrender and fully immerse themselves in the experience.

Now, dear reader, it is time for you to unleash your creativity and touch the lives of others through the power of Yoga Nidra scripting. Let your words become an instrument of healing and growth. May your journey be filled with joy, abundance, and endless discoveries as you continue to explore the depths of this ancient practice.
Best wishes on your writing and teaching endeavors, and may your Yoga Nidra scripts illuminate the path for countless individuals. Happy writing!"

ADDITIONAL RESOURCES

Books

Feuerstein, Georg. 1998. The Yoga Tradition: Its History, Literature, Philosophy and Practice. Hohm Press, London

Saraswati, Swami Satyananda. 1984. Yoga Nidra. Bihar School of Yoga

Richard Miller, 2005, Yoga Nidra, The Meditative Heart of Yoga. Sounds True, Colorado

Swami Jyotirmayananda. 1973. Meditate the Tantric Yoga Way. Lillian K. Donat

Nrusingh Charan Panda. 2004. Yoga-Nidra (Yogic Trance) Theory, practice and applications. D.K. Print World Ltd

Sites
www.yoganidranetwork.org/nidras/
www.swamij.com/yoga-nidra-method1.htm

This guide was written by

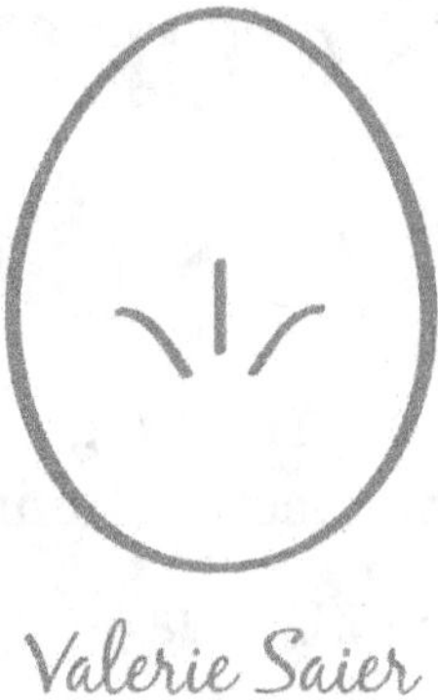

Find more at
www.nlpsynplus.com